DOCTOR DEATH

The Harrowing Tale of Harold Shipman,

one of the Most Prolific Serial Killers in

Modern Medical History

By

Heather B. Eldredge

Copyright @2023

TABLE OF CONTENT

Harold Shipman, a British physician, gained notoriety for leading a terrifying double life as both a respected doctor and a serial killer. Shipman, born on January 14, 1946 in Nottingham, England, initially made a name for himself as a dedicated and empathetic family doctor. He earned the respect and admiration of both his patients and colleagues. However, beneath that seemingly pleasant exterior lurked a sinister and malevolent individual. For decades, Shipman exploited his position of trust to prey on vulnerable patients, primarily targeting older women, and ultimately causing their deaths.

Shipman would give his patients false diagnoses of ailments before administering a fatal dose of diamorphine. Between 1975 and 1998, approximately 250 victims visited Harold Shipman's office, unknowingly meeting their tragic fate.

His ability to conceal his horrible actions under a mask of sympathy and love remains a haunting reminder of the lowest depths of human deception. The dark legacy of "Doctor Death" has sparked discussions on patient safety, medical ethics, and the abuse of power and trust by individuals in positions of authority.

CHAPTER ONE

Early Life of Harold Shipman

Harold Frederick Shipman, commonly referred to as "Fred," was born on January 14, 1946, as the middle child in a working-class family. Vera, his mother, exhibited a high degree of control. As a teenager, he became a social outcast due to the superiority complex that had been instilled in him from a young age.

He diligently took care of his mother after she was diagnosed with terminal lung cancer. Despite the difficult circumstances, he remained positive and provided her with the best possible care until she peacefully passed away on June 21, 1963. He was fascinated by the relief that morphine brought to her pain. After failing his entry examinations for medical school, the first time, he was determined to try again. The passing of his mother served as inspiration, and two years later, he commenced his medical studies at Leeds University. Primrose was the woman who would become his wife, and he met her while he was still a loner. They got married when she was 17 and he was 19 and had their first child.

In 1974, he had two children and was employed as a family doctor in Todmorden, Yorkshire. During this time, it seems that he developed an addiction to the opioid medication known as Pethidine. In 1975, he made the decision to join a drug rehabilitation center. This choice came after his fellow doctors discovered that he had been forging prescriptions for large amounts of the substance. Following a thorough investigation, he was determined to be guilty of forgery and subsequently received a minor fine.

After a few years, Shipman became a part of the team at Hyde's Donneybrook

Medical Centre. Despite his junior colleagues perceiving him as arrogant, he was able to gain the respect of both patients and colleagues due to his exceptional skills. He had been employed there for almost twenty years, yet his peculiar behavior went largely unnoticed by those in the medical field.

The Crimes of Doctor Shipman

Shipman's first patient was Eva Lyons, a 70-year-old woman, in March 1975. It was the evening before the day that was special to her. Although Shipman's addiction was not discovered until the following year, he had already accumulated a sufficient amount of diamorphine to cause the deaths of hundreds of individuals. Despite being sacked for prescription forgery, Shipman was not expelled from the ranks of the General Medical Council, the regulatory body for doctors. He received a cautionary letter.

According to investigators, Shipman would often take breaks and then resume his killing spree during his decades of terror. However, his technique for committing murder never changed. The victims of his crimes spanned a wide range of ages, from 93-year-old Anne Cooper to 41-year-old Peter Lewis. It is important to note that all of these individuals were vulnerable and lacked the ability to defend themselves. He would either watch them die or send them home to die after administering a fatal dose of diamorphine.

The local undertaker discovered that the majority of Dr. Shipman's patients were fully clothed and in a consistent position, either sitting up or lying on a sofa, at the time of their passing. Due to his concerns, he immediately approached Shipman, who reassured him that everything was fine. Dr. Susan Booth, a concerned physician, discovered the worrisome similarities and promptly alerted the local coroner's office. Subsequently, the coroner's office contacted the police to investigate the matter.

Shipman was exonerated after a confidential investigation uncovered that his paperwork was in order. The investigation failed to consider important sources of information about Shipman's past, such as the General Medical Council and criminal records. Upon further investigation, it was discovered that Shipman had manipulated the medical records of his patients in order to provide false evidence supporting the causes of their deaths.

The police inquiry failed to consider Shipman's criminal history. If they had contacted the medical board and requested his record, they might have discovered that he had previously falsified prescriptions. Shipman has taken additional measures to hide his actions by falsifying medical diagnoses for his victims. As a result, the investigation revealed no suspicious activities, enabling the doctor to continue their dangerous actions without facing any consequences.

Shipman vehemently denied all claims, thereby making it exceedingly difficult to ascertain the exact timeline of when he initially started killing his patients or the precise number of individuals who lost their lives due to his actions. He concealed himself using his reputation as a caring family doctor.

CHAPTER TWO

Mayor Kathleen's Murder

Angela Woodruff, the daughter of one of his victims, refused to accept the official account of her mother's murder. Her determination ultimately led to the cessation of his killing spree.

Shipman's attempt to forge the will of Kathleen Grundy, an 81-year-old victim and former mayor of Hyde, ultimately led to the exposure of his wrongdoings. The body of 81-year-old widow Kathleen Grundy was discovered at her house on June 24, 1998, following a visit by Shipman. Shipman selected the "cremation" option mentioned in Grundy's will in order to hide the truth that he had administered a lethal dose of diamorphine to her. Afterward, he utilized the typewriter to exclude her relatives entirely from the will, ensuring that he would inherit all of the assets. Shipman informed Woodruff that an autopsy was deemed unnecessary. Consequently, Grundy's body was cremated and buried as per the instructions provided by her daughter. However, the local solicitors notified Angela Woodruff, Grundy's daughter, about the will after her burial. She immediately noticed that something was wrong and promptly contacted the authorities.

Woodruff, a lawyer who had always managed her mother's affairs, was shocked to discover that another will existed, which left the majority of her mother's assets to Dr. Shipman. Woodruff was convinced that Shipman had committed the murder of her mother and subsequently fabricated the will in order to exploit the financial benefits resulting from her demise. After notifying the authorities, Detective Superintendent Bernard Postles reviewed the material and reached the same conclusion.

The postmortem examination of Grundy's body revealed that she had overdosed on morphine three hours prior to her death, which coincided with Shipman's visit. In the following two months, an additional 11 victims' bodies were found. Authorities also investigated the computer at Shipman's clinic. They discovered that the doctor had created fraudulent records to support the false causes of death he had listed for his victims. Shipman argued that Grundy was dependent on opiates such as morphine or heroin, providing his own notes as evidence to support his claim. Additionally, Shipman contended that this dependency existed simultaneously. However, after her death, detectives were able to determine that Shipman was indeed the author of the notes that were discovered on his computer. During the search of Shipman's house, investigators discovered several noteworthy items. These included medical records, an intriguing jewelry collection, and an antique typewriter. It was later determined that the typewriter had been used to create Grundy's forged will. Upon examining the medical records that were confiscated, the police swiftly deduced that this particular case encompassed more than just the initially reported death. They promptly focused their attention on cases where the victims had not been cremated and had passed away subsequent to Shipman's visits to their residences. The police subsequently verified an additional 14 cases in which Shipman deliberately caused the deaths of patients by administering lethal doses of diamorphine. He then proceeded to falsify their death certificates and medical records, creating the illusion that these patients were already in critical condition prior to their demise.

Shipman had convinced families in multiple instances to cremate their loved ones without conducting any additional investigation into the circumstances surrounding their deaths. This includes cases where the cause of death was unknown. Shipman would provide electronic medical records as evidence to support his claims when people questioned his declarations about the causes of death.

CHAPTER THREE

The Investigation, Trial and Its Aftermath

The police discovered that Shipman would frequently alter medical records soon after murdering a patient, in order to align his narrative with the official documentation. Shipman overlooked the fact that the computer would automatically record the time of any modifications made to the files. As a result, it became effortless for law enforcement to determine which files had been tampered with. Despite being interviewed by the police and criminal psychiatrists, Harold Shipman continued to deny the murders. He declined to open his eyes, let out a yawn, and remained composed as the police interrogated him and presented him with images of his victims. Shipman was initially charged with 15 killings by the police; however, it is widely believed that he may have been responsible for the deaths of anywhere between 250 and 450 individuals.

On September 7, 1998, the police formally accused Shipman of 15 counts of murder and one count of forgery. This accusation came after an extensive investigation, which involved multiple exhumations and examinations.

The trial against Shipman began on October 5, 1999, at Preston Crown Court. The defense team's motion to divide the trial into three parts, specifically focusing on cases involving physical evidence, cases without physical evidence, and the Grundy case which stands out due to the forgery, was unsuccessful. Additionally, their attempts to exclude damaging evidence related to Shipman's fraudulent accumulation of morphine and other drugs were also unsuccessful. As a result, the trial proceeded with all 16 charges listed in the indictment.

According to the prosecution, Shipman allegedly killed 15 patients due to his desire to exert control over their lives and have the ultimate authority. They also mentioned that he lacked compassion as none of his victims were in the later stages of their lives.

Woodruff was the first witness to testify. The jurors were pleased by her candor and her story of her determined pursuit of the truth. The defense's attempts to discredit her were unsuccessful. The government pathologist presented the post mortem findings to the court, revealing that the leading cause of death was morphine poisoning. The findings were quite grisly. The subsequent examination of the fabricated will revealed that Grundy had never touched it, and a handwriting expert determined that her signature was a poorly executed forgery. According to the testimony of a police computer analyst, Shipman was found to have manipulated his electronic patient files.

This manipulation typically occurred shortly after the patients' deaths, with the intention of falsely indicating the presence of symptoms that were not actually present. As the trial progressed and testimonies from the loved ones of Shipman's other victims were presented, a more comprehensive understanding of Shipman's pattern of actions began to surface. Not only did he lack compassion for his patients and disregard the wishes of their family members, but he also refused to attempt a revival. To make matters worse, it was later discovered that he would feign calling 911 in front of grieving loved ones, only to abruptly end the call upon realizing that the patient had already passed away. There is clear evidence in the phone company's records that no calls were actually made.

Finally, evidence was presented that revealed his drug hoarding activities. This included instances where he falsely prescribed morphine to patients who did not require it, as well as cases where he excessively prescribed morphine to those who did need it. Additionally, it was discovered that he would visit the homes of the recently deceased to "dispose" of their surplus medication.

Shipman's arrogant behavior during the trial hindered his defense's ability to portray him as a compassionate and knowledgeable medical expert. Despite their attempts to win over the jurors, his excessive arrogance and numerous stories prevented them from being deceived by his obvious lies.

After a comprehensive summary provided by the judge and a reminder to the jury that there were no eyewitnesses to Shipman's acts of killing his patients, the jury reached a unanimous verdict of guilty on all charges on the afternoon of January 31, 2000. There were 15 murder charges and one forgery charge. The judge removed the possibility of parole for all fifteen inmates who had been sentenced to life, and he changed the four-year forgery term to a "whole life" sentence. Shipman was incarcerated at Durham Institution.

The medical community was shocked by the news of a doctor who had killed 15 patients. However, further investigations into his case list history revealed that this information was largely insignificant. Professor Richard Baker from the University of Leicester conducted a clinical audit to compare the quantity and pattern of deaths in Shipman's practice with those of other doctors. Shipman was present during a significantly higher number of deaths, and the mortality rates were notably higher among his elderly patients. The investigation has concluded that, spanning a period of 24 years, he may have been responsible for the deaths of at least 236 individuals.

A separate commission, headed by High Court Judge Dame Janet Smith, conducted an investigation into the deaths of 500 patients under Shipman's care. Their extensive 2,000-page report concluded that there was a strong likelihood that he had murdered at least 218 of his patients. However, Dame Janet provided this number as an estimate rather than a precise calculation due to certain cases lacking sufficient evidence to ensure certainty. The report suggested that Shipman may have had a compulsion for killing and criticized the police investigation processes. It pointed out that the lack of experience among the investigating officers resulted in missed opportunities to bring Shipman to court earlier. The first potential victim of the individual in question could be Margaret Thompson, a 67-year-old woman who passed away in March 1971 while in the process of recovering from a stroke. It is worth noting that this incident occurred just a few months after he obtained his medical license. However, it is important to mention that no deaths prior to 1975 have been officially confirmed as being connected to him.

Without a precise number, Shipman's status as a British patient killer was quickly elevated to that of the world's most prolific known serial killer, thanks to the sheer magnitude of his deadly operations. While incarcerated in Durham Prison, he steadfastly maintained his innocence, receiving unwavering support from his wife, Primrose, and their family.

CHAPTER FOUR

Death and Legacy of Doctor Death

In the year 2000, Shipman was sentenced to life in prison without the possibility of parole. He was transferred from Manchester Prison to Wakefield Prison in West Yorkshire, where he tragically took his own life. On January 13, 2004, Shipman was found hanging in his cell, just one day before his 58th birthday. He had previously confided in his probation officer about his contemplation of suicide, with the intention of leaving his entire estate to his wife in a single lump sum payment. We will never know the reason behind his actions now that he is no longer with us. One of the suggested explanations for Shipman's murderous impulses is that he sought revenge for his mother's death. Others, taking a more sympathetic stance, argue that he administered diamorphine to the elderly with good intentions. Some people argue that the doctor's need to demonstrate his ability to take lives, in addition to saving them, was due to his God complex.

There are conflicting reports regarding the whereabouts of his body. According to some sources, his body is still in a Sheffield morgue. However, there are also claims that his family has custody of his body due to suspicions of foul play in his cell. They are reportedly waiting to bury him until additional testing has been conducted.

The legacy of Harold Shipman is characterized by feelings of dread, immense loss of life, and a profound sense of betrayal. He may have killed over 200 patients, and the exact number may never be determined, which has earned him a notorious reputation as one of the most infamous serial killers in history. The regulations and medical education standards in the UK were altered due to his criminal behavior. The families affected by Shipman's cruel and horrific actions are left with the enduring pain of losing a loved one, a loss from which they may never fully recover. It is often difficult for individuals to comprehend how someone who is responsible for their well-being could commit such a heinous act. The scandal that rocked the medical community has caused patients across the country to lose trust in doctors. Shipman's crimes had a significant impact on the judicial system, leading to the implementation of new regulations regarding the investigation and documentation of medical deaths. His actions prompted a public investigation, which ultimately resulted in recommendations to improve communication between medical experts and reform medical regulation.

Shipman's conviction has made his story a prominent example of the dangers associated with the abuse of power in the medical field and has contributed to the study of criminal psychology. Although his atrocities will forever be remembered with infamy, it is crucial that we continue our efforts to learn from them in order to prevent their repetition.

How to Protect Elderly Family Members from Abuse

Harold Shipman's tragic tale serves as a frightening reminder that even the most vulnerable members of society can be abused by those entrusted with their care. As our aging relatives demand more care and help, it is critical to put safeguards in place to protect them from harm.

Extensive background checks:

Conducting thorough background checks is an important part in the decision process when hiring in-home caregivers or contemplating a senior living facility. Seek out reliable agencies with a track record of excellent caregiving experiences, and double-check possible caregivers' credentials and references.

Maintain Consistent Communication:

It is critical to maintain open and regular communication with both the elderly relative and their carers. Engage with your loved one on a regular basis, either in person or by phone or video calls, to be updated about their well-being. Develop a relationship with their caretakers and encourage them to immediately report any concerns or changes in the senior's status.

Educate and Empower Your Elderly Family Member:

It is critical to educate your senior loved one about their rights and the warning signs of abuse. Make it clear to them that they can contact you or other trusted individuals if they ever feel uncomfortable or dangerous. Empowering kids with information can help prevent abuse and encourage them to speak up if something doesn't feel right.

Keep an eye out for warning signs:

Recognizing potential misuse red flags is critical. Keep an eye out for physical signals such unexplained bruises, wounds, or weight loss, as well as emotional signs like unexpected changes in behavior or fearfulness around specific people. Financial exploitation is another issue to be concerned about, so keep an eye out for any strange transactions or abnormalities in their financial records.

Visit Frequently:

Frequent visits to your elderly relative not only provide them with emotional support, but also allow you to examine their living conditions and interactions with carers. Unexpected visits can help you assess the level of care they receive while they are not being monitored.

Encourage Social Participation:

Isolation might increase an elderly person's vulnerability to abuse. Encourage your loved one to participate in social activities, groups, or community events to give them a sense of belonging and to limit their exposure to possible abusers.

Any Suspected Abuse Should Be Reported:

Act promptly if you suspect mistreatment or neglect. Inform the proper authorities, such as adult protective services or law enforcement, of your concerns. Your prompt action can protect not only your loved one, but also others in similar situations.

Conclusion:

Elder abuse prevention necessitates a proactive approach that includes vigilance, communication, and education. By taking these important actions, we may protect our older relatives from danger and guarantee that their golden years are filled with the care, respect, and love they deserve. We can work together to establish an atmosphere where elders are safeguarded and valued, free from those who would betray their confidence and cause harm.

END